The Total Body Workout Guide:
Get Fit and Stay in Shape

Adam Edward

Copyright

Table of content

Introduction to a total body workout

A total body workout is a type of exercise routine that targets all major muscle groups in the body. This type of workout is an excellent way to improve overall strength, endurance, and flexibility. A total body workout can be done using bodyweight exercises, resistance training, or a combination of both.

The benefits of a total body workout are numerous. By working all major muscle groups, you can improve your overall body composition, increase muscle tone, and burn calories more efficiently. This type of workout is also great for improving cardiovascular health and reducing the risk of chronic diseases like heart disease, diabetes, and obesity.

When planning a total body workout, it's important to focus on exercises that work multiple muscle groups at once. Compound exercises like squats, deadlifts, lunges, and push-ups are great examples of exercises that work several muscle groups simultaneously. Isolation exercises like bicep curls and tricep extensions can be added as supplemental exercises, but they should not be the focus of the workout.

It's also important to vary the intensity of the workout to challenge the body and prevent plateaus. This can be done by increasing the weight or resistance used, increasing the number of reps or sets, or reducing the rest time between exercises.

In addition to resistance training, a total body workout should also include cardiovascular exercise. This can be done by incorporating activities like running, cycling, or jumping jacks into the workout. The amount of cardiovascular exercise needed will depend on individual fitness goals, but a good rule of thumb is to aim for at least 20-30 minutes of moderate to intense cardio per session.

Before starting any new exercise program, it's important to consult with a healthcare professional and get clearance to exercise. This is especially important if you have any pre-existing medical conditions or injuries.

In summary, a total body workout is an effective way to improve overall fitness and health. By incorporating compound exercises and cardiovascular training into your routine, you can work all major muscle groups and burn calories more efficiently. However, it's important to vary the intensity of the workout and seek clearance from a healthcare professional before starting any new exercise program.

When designing a total body workout, it's important to create a balanced routine that targets all muscle groups equally. This means including exercises that work the upper body, lower body, and core muscles. It's also important to include exercises that work both the pushing and pulling movements to ensure balanced muscle development.

To ensure the effectiveness of the total body workout, it's important to have proper form and technique for each exercise. This will not only prevent injuries but also maximize the benefits of each exercise. It's recommended to start with a weight or resistance that is challenging but manageable, and gradually increase the weight or resistance as you progress.

A total body workout can be done in a variety of settings, including at home, in a gym, or outdoors.

Bodyweight exercises like squats, lunges, push-ups, and planks can be done anywhere without the need for equipment. Resistance training can be done using dumbbells, resistance bands, or weight machines at a gym.

In addition to resistance and cardiovascular exercise, it's also important to incorporate flexibility training into a total body workout. Stretching exercises like yoga or static stretches can help improve range of motion, reduce the risk of injury, and aid in muscle recovery.

It's important to have a balanced approach to fitness and not rely solely on one type of exercise. A total body workout should be complemented with a healthy diet, adequate sleep, and stress management techniques to achieve overall well-being.

In conclusion, a total body workout is an excellent way to improve overall fitness, strength, and flexibility. By incorporating compound exercises, cardiovascular training, and flexibility exercises, you can work all major muscle groups and improve your overall health. It's important to have proper form and technique, vary the intensity of the workout, and seek clearance from a healthcare

professional before starting any new exercise
program.

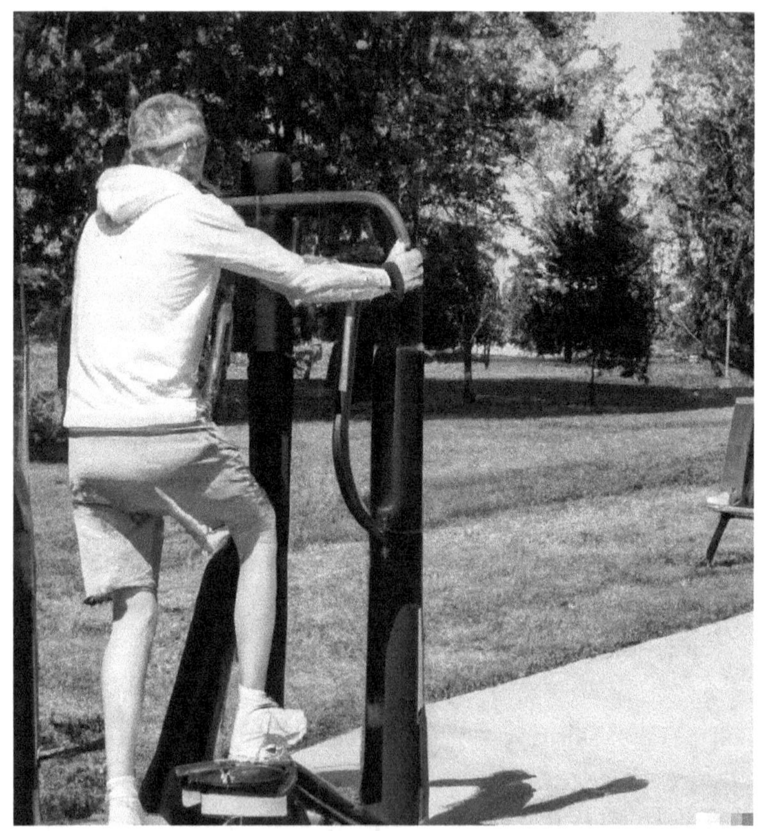

The benefits of a total body workout

A total body workout is a form of exercise that targets all the major muscle groups of the body, including the arms, legs, chest, back, shoulders, and core. It is a highly effective way to improve overall fitness and health, and can provide numerous benefits for individuals of all ages and fitness levels.

One of the most significant benefits of a total body workout is improved cardiovascular health. This type of exercise increases heart rate, which improves blood flow and oxygen delivery to the muscles. This can reduce the risk of heart disease, stroke, and other cardiovascular problems.

In addition to cardiovascular benefits, a total body workout can also help to build and maintain lean muscle mass. By engaging multiple muscle groups at once, it can help to increase muscle strength and endurance, which can enhance overall physical performance and reduce the risk of injury.

Another important benefit of a total body workout is improved flexibility and mobility. By incorporating stretching and mobility exercises into the workout routine, individuals can improve joint mobility, range of motion, and overall flexibility, which can enhance athletic performance and reduce the risk of injury.

A total body workout can also provide mental health benefits. Exercise has been shown to reduce stress, anxiety, and depression, and can improve overall mood and mental well-being. By engaging in a regular total body workout routine, individuals can reduce the risk of developing mental health problems and improve overall quality of life.

Finally, a total body workout can help to improve overall body composition. By burning calories and increasing muscle mass, it can help to reduce body fat and improve overall body composition. This can lead to improved physical appearance and enhanced self-confidence.

Overall, a total body workout is a highly effective way to improve overall fitness and health. It can provide numerous benefits, including improved cardiovascular health, increased muscle strength and endurance, improved flexibility and mobility, and enhanced mental well-being. By incorporating a total body workout into a regular exercise routine, individuals can improve overall quality of life and enjoy long-term health benefits

One of the advantages of a total body workout is that it can be done with minimal equipment, making it accessible and affordable for everyone. It can be performed at home, in a gym, or even outdoors with bodyweight exercises. This makes it a convenient and practical way to stay active and healthy.

Furthermore, a total body workout can be tailored to meet the specific needs and goals of individuals. Whether the goal is to lose weight, build muscle, improve cardiovascular fitness, or simply maintain overall health, a total body workout can be customized to meet those needs.

Incorporating a total body workout into a regular exercise routine can also help to prevent plateaus in fitness progress. By regularly challenging the body with new exercises and increasing the intensity of the workout, individuals can continue to see improvements in their fitness levels over time.

Additionally, a total body workout can help to improve sports performance. Many sports require the use of multiple muscle groups, and a total body workout can help to develop those muscles and improve overall athletic ability.

Lastly, a total body workout can provide a sense of accomplishment and satisfaction. Completing a challenging workout can boost confidence and improve overall self-esteem. This can translate into other areas of life, such as work and relationships, and can help to create a more positive outlook on life.

In conclusion, the benefits of a total body workout are numerous and far-reaching. It can improve cardiovascular health, build and maintain muscle mass, improve flexibility and mobility, enhance mental well-being, improve body composition, and much more. By incorporating a total body workout into a regular exercise routine, individuals can enjoy improved overall health, fitness, and quality of life.

Essential exercises for a full body workout

A full body workout is an excellent way to maintain overall health and fitness. Engaging in regular exercise has numerous benefits such as weight loss, improved heart health, increased muscle mass, and a stronger immune system. The following are some essential exercises that you can incorporate into your full body workout routine:

Squats: Squats are a compound exercise that engages multiple muscles in your body. They target your quadriceps, hamstrings, glutes, and core muscles. Squats can be performed using your body weight or with added resistance such as a barbell or dumbbell.

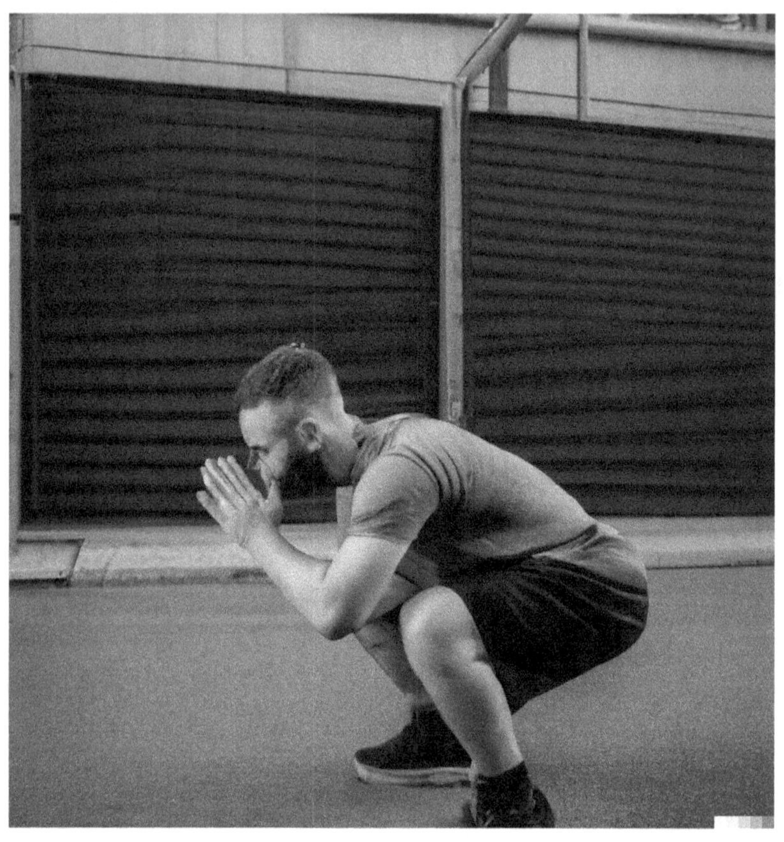

Lunges: Lunges are another excellent compound exercise that targets your glutes, hamstrings, and quads. They can be done with or without weights and can be modified to make them more challenging.

Deadlifts: Deadlifts are a great exercise for building overall strength and mass in your lower body. They primarily target your hamstrings, glutes, and lower back muscles. Deadlifts can be done with a barbell or dumbbells.

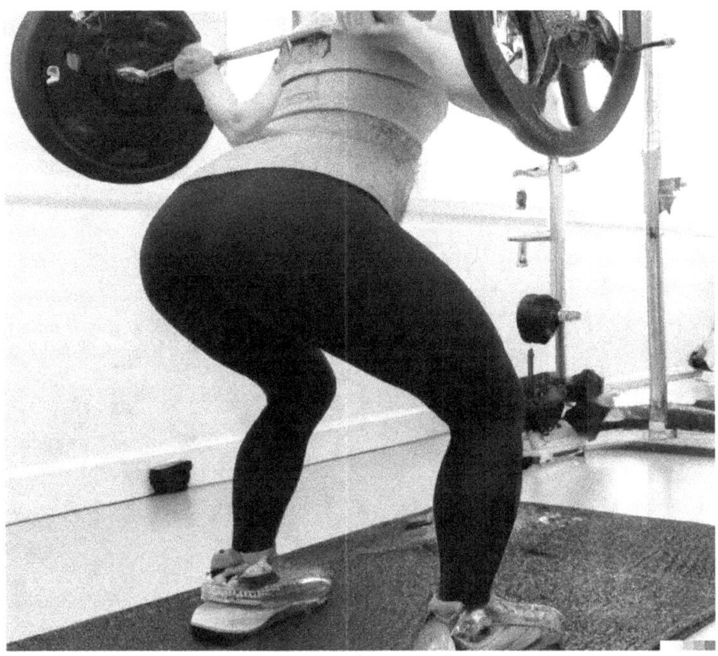

Bench Press: The bench press is an excellent compound exercise that targets your chest, shoulders, and triceps. It is a great exercise for building upper body strength and can be performed using a barbell or dumbbells.

Pull-Ups: Pull-ups are a challenging exercise that targets your back, biceps, and forearms. They can be done using a pull-up bar or assisted with resistance bands.

Push-Ups: Push-ups are a classic exercise that targets your chest, shoulders, and triceps. They can be done using your body weight or modified to make them more challenging.

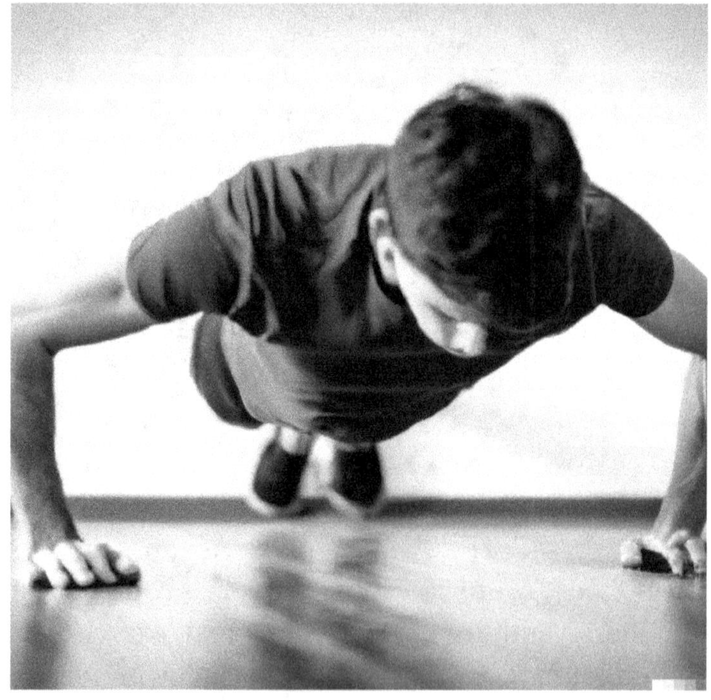

Planks: Planks are a great exercise for building core strength and stability. They target your abs, back, and glutes. Planks can be performed in various positions, such as the traditional plank, side plank, and reverse plank.

Burpees: Burpees are a full-body exercise that engages your chest, shoulders, triceps, abs, back, and legs. They are a great exercise for building overall fitness and endurance.

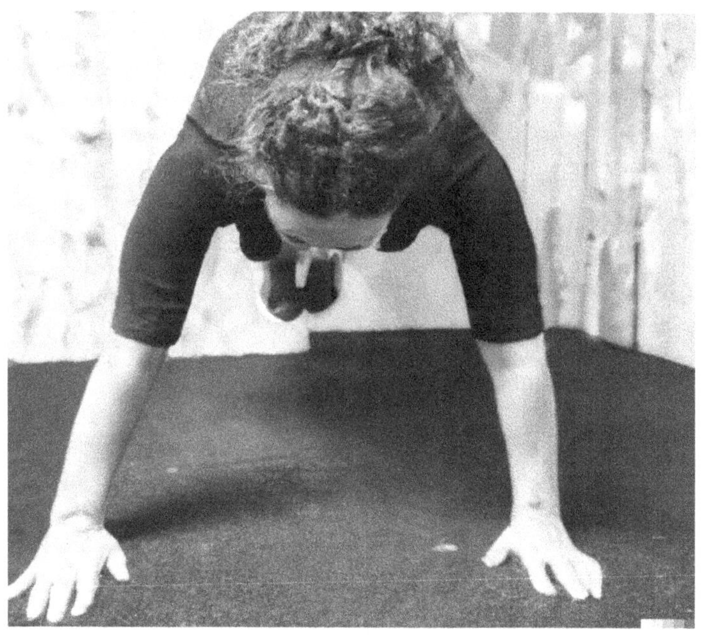

Jumping Jacks: Jumping jacks are a simple yet effective exercise that engages your whole body. They are a great way to warm up before a workout or to get your heart rate up during a cardio session.

Bicycle Crunches: Bicycle crunches are a great exercise for targeting your abs and obliques. They can help to strengthen your core muscles and improve your posture. To perform this exercise, lie on your back with your hands behind your head and lift your legs off the ground. Bring your left knee towards your right elbow while extending your right leg. Then switch sides, bringing your right knee towards your left elbow while extending your left leg.

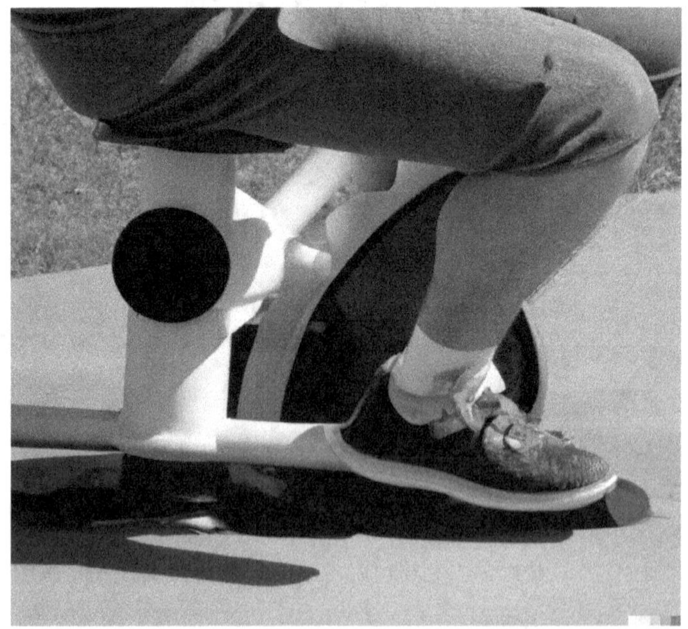

Romanian Deadlifts: Romanian deadlifts are a variation of the deadlift that focus on your hamstrings and glutes. They can be performed using a barbell or dumbbells. To perform this exercise, stand with your feet shoulder-width apart and hold the barbell or dumbbells in front of your thighs. Hinge at your hips and lower the weight towards the ground while keeping your back straight. Return to the starting position by squeezing your glutes and hamstrings.

Overhead Press: The overhead press is a great exercise for building upper body strength and targeting your shoulders, triceps, and upper back muscles. It can be performed using a barbell or dumbbells. To perform this exercise, stand with your feet shoulder-width apart and hold the weight at shoulder height. Press the weight overhead while keeping your core engaged and your back straight.

Dips: Dips are a great exercise for targeting your chest, triceps, and shoulders. They can be performed using parallel bars or a bench. To perform this exercise, start by placing your hands on the bars or bench behind you and lowering your body until your arms are at a 90-degree angle. Then push yourself back up to the starting position by engaging your chest and triceps.

Box Jumps: Box jumps are a great plyometric exercise that can help to improve your explosive power and leg strength. They can be performed using a box or step. To perform this exercise, start by standing in front of the box with your feet shoulder-width apart. Jump onto the box while landing softly on the balls of your feet. Then step down and repeat.

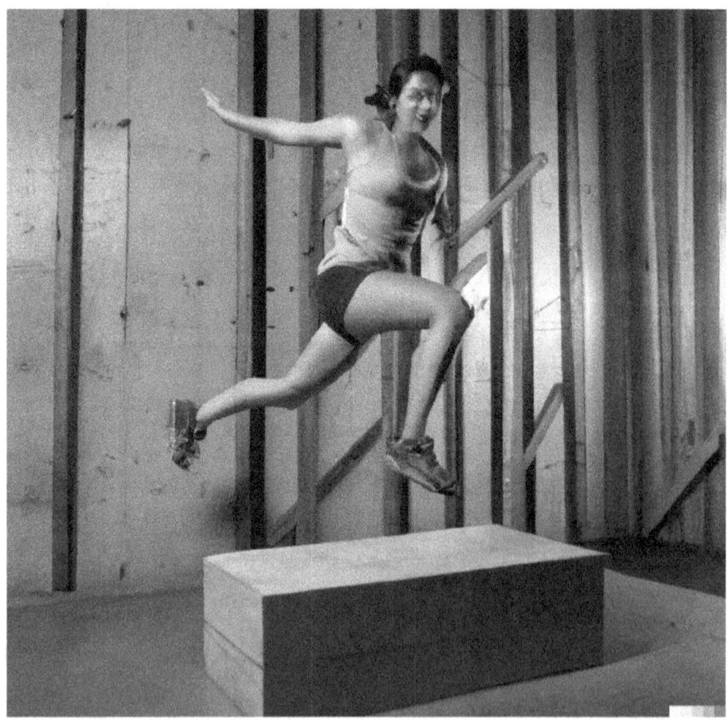

Farmer's Walk: The farmer's walk is a great exercise for improving your grip strength, core stability, and overall strength. It can be performed using heavy dumbbells or kettlebells. To perform this exercise, pick up the weights and walk forward while keeping your core engaged and your shoulders back.

Box Squats: Box squats are a variation of the squat that can help to improve your squat form and build lower body strength. They can be performed using a box or bench. To perform this exercise, start by standing in front of the box with your feet shoulder-width apart. Sit back onto the box while keeping your back straight and your knees in line with your toes. Then stand back up to the starting position.

Chin-Ups: Chin-ups are a great exercise for targeting your back, biceps, and forearms. They can be performed using a pull-up bar or assisted with resistance bands. To perform this exercise, start by hanging from the bar with your palms facing towards you. Pull your body up until your chin is above the bar, then lower yourself back down.

Kettlebell Swings: Kettlebell swings are a full-body exercise that can help to improve your strength, power, and endurance. They primarily target your glutes, hamstrings, and core muscles. To perform this exercise, start by standing with your feet shoulder-width apart and holding the kettlebell with both hands. Hinge at your hips and swing the kettlebell between your legs, then explosively swing it up to shoulder height.

Inverted Rows: Inverted rows are a great exercise for targeting your back, biceps, and core muscles. They can be performed using a bar or TRX straps. To perform this exercise, start by lying underneath the bar or TRX straps and holding onto them with your hands. Pull your chest up towards the bar or straps while keeping your core engaged and your shoulders back.

Battle Ropes: Battle ropes are a great cardio exercise that can also help to build upper body strength and endurance. They can be performed using heavy ropes or resistance bands. To perform this exercise, start by holding onto the ropes or bands with both hands and moving them up and down in a rapid, alternating motion.

In conclusion, a full body workout routine that incorporates these essential exercises can help you achieve overall fitness and health. It is essential to vary your exercises to prevent boredom and maximize your results. Always remember to consult with a fitness professional before beginning any exercise program to ensure safety and effectiveness.

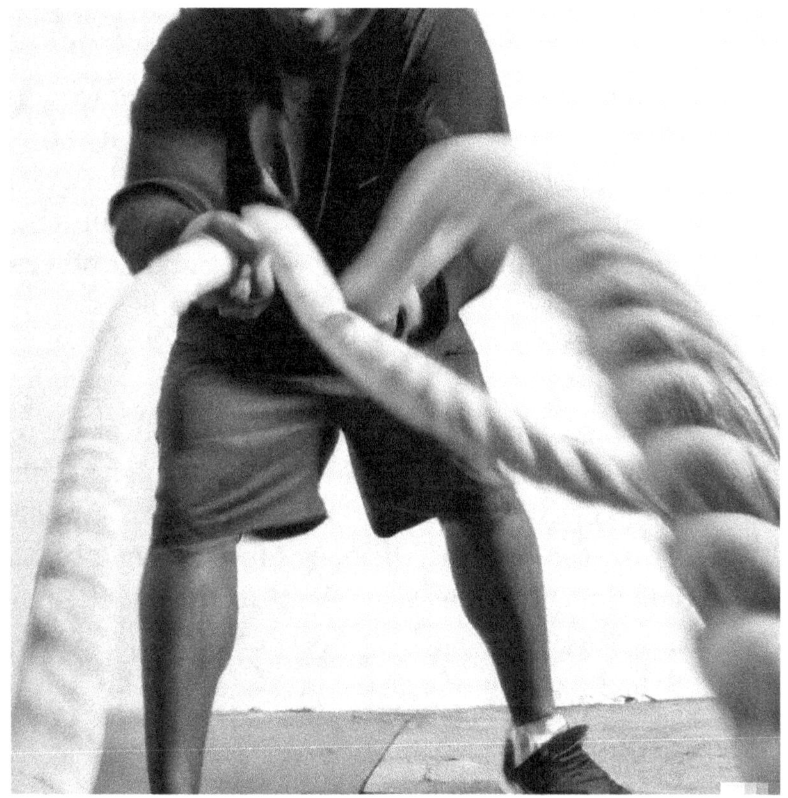

The importance of cardio in a total body workout

Cardiovascular exercise, commonly known as cardio, is any form of physical activity that increases heart rate and works the cardiovascular system. It includes activities such as running, cycling, swimming, dancing, and many others. Cardio is an essential part of a total body workout, and here's why:

Cardiovascular health: Regular cardio exercise is crucial for maintaining good cardiovascular health. Cardio helps to strengthen the heart muscle, increase the heart's efficiency, and improve blood circulation. By doing so, it helps to reduce the risk of heart diseases such as heart attack, stroke, and high blood pressure.

Weight management: Cardio is also an excellent way to manage weight. When you perform cardio, you burn calories and fat, which can help you to lose weight or maintain a healthy weight. This is because cardio exercises increase your metabolic rate, which means your body burns more calories even when you're not exercising.

Increased endurance: Cardio is an effective way to improve endurance and stamina. When you do cardio exercises regularly, you increase the amount of oxygen that your body can use during exercise. This, in turn, helps to improve your endurance and allows you to perform physical activities for longer periods without feeling tired.

Improved mental health: Cardio is also good for your mental health. Exercise releases endorphins, which are chemicals in the brain that promote feelings of happiness and well-being. Regular cardio exercise can help to reduce stress, anxiety, and depression and improve your overall mood.

Improved immune system: Cardio has been shown to improve the immune system's function by increasing the production of white blood cells, which help to fight off infections and diseases.

Enhanced athletic performance: Cardio is essential for athletes and individuals who participate in sports. It helps to improve endurance, speed, and agility, which are all critical factors in athletic performance.

Varied workout routine: Adding cardio to your total body workout can also help to keep your workouts interesting and varied. This can help to prevent boredom and keep you motivated to continue your fitness journey.

In conclusion, cardio is a crucial component of a total body workout. It provides numerous health benefits, including improved cardiovascular health, weight management, increased endurance, improved mental health, improved immune system, enhanced athletic performance, and varied workout routines. By incorporating cardio into your fitness routine, you can achieve a well-rounded and balanced approach to fitness and enjoy a healthier and happier lifestyle.

The role of strength training in a total body workout

Strength training is a type of physical exercise that is designed to increase muscular strength and endurance. It involves the use of weights or resistance bands to challenge the muscles and improve overall fitness. When it comes to a total body workout, strength training plays a crucial role in improving overall health and fitness.

Strength training has several benefits that are essential for a total body workout. Firstly, it increases muscle strength, which is essential for performing daily activities such as lifting, carrying, and pushing. It also improves bone density, reducing the risk of osteoporosis and fractures.

In addition to this, strength training can help to improve body composition by reducing body fat and increasing muscle mass. This can help to increase metabolism, burn calories and maintain a healthy weight. It also helps to improve muscle endurance, making it easier to perform physical activities for longer periods of time.

Strength training also has mental health benefits. It can help to reduce stress levels, improve mood and increase self-esteem. It also helps to improve sleep quality, which is essential for overall health and wellbeing.

When it comes to a total body workout, strength training should be incorporated as a key component. This can be achieved through a variety of exercises that target different muscle groups. For example, compound exercises such as squats, deadlifts, and bench presses target multiple muscle groups at once, making them ideal for a total body workout.

It is important to note that strength training should be performed correctly and safely to avoid injury. This can be achieved by using proper form and technique, starting with lighter weights and gradually increasing the weight as you become stronger, and taking adequate rest between sets.

Incorporating strength training into a total body workout can also help to prevent injury and improve performance in other forms of exercise, such as cardiovascular exercise and sports. Stronger muscles provide greater stability and support for the joints, reducing the risk of injury during physical activity. Additionally, improved muscle strength and endurance can lead to improved performance in other forms of exercise, allowing individuals to work out for longer periods of time and with greater intensity.

It is important to note that strength training should not be the only component of a total body workout. Other forms of exercise, such as cardiovascular exercise and flexibility training, should also be incorporated to achieve a well-rounded workout routine. This can help to improve overall fitness and reduce the risk of injury.

When designing a total body workout that incorporates strength training, it is important to consider individual goals and fitness level. Beginners may want to start with bodyweight exercises or lighter weights, while more advanced individuals may want to incorporate heavier weights or more complex exercises. Consulting with a certified personal trainer can also be helpful in developing a safe and effective strength training program.

Moreover, strength training is an essential component of a total body workout. It offers numerous physical and mental health benefits and can help to prevent injury and improve performance in other forms of exercise. By incorporating strength training into a well-rounded workout routine, individuals can achieve their fitness goals and improve overall health and wellbeing.

In conclusion, strength training plays a crucial role in a total body workout. It has several benefits that improve overall health and fitness, and it should be incorporated as a key component in any workout routine. By using proper form and technique and taking adequate rest between sets, strength training can help to improve muscle strength, endurance, body composition, and mental health.

Resistance training for a total body workout

Resistance training is a type of exercise that focuses on building muscular strength and endurance by using external resistance, such as weights, resistance bands, or bodyweight. Resistance training is often used as part of a total body workout program to help individuals achieve their fitness goals.

The benefits of resistance training for a total body workout are numerous. It helps to build muscle mass, increase bone density, improve body composition, boost metabolism, and enhance overall physical performance. Additionally, resistance training can help prevent or manage chronic diseases, such as type 2 diabetes, osteoporosis, and heart disease.

A total body workout that incorporates resistance training typically includes exercises that target all major muscle groups, including the chest, back, legs, shoulders, arms, and core. Some examples of resistance training exercises that can be included in a total body workout program are:

Squats: This exercise targets the legs, glutes, and core. It can be performed with weights or bodyweight.

Deadlifts: This exercise targets the legs, back, and core. It can be performed with weights or bodyweight.

Push-ups: This exercise targets the chest, shoulders, triceps, and core. It can be performed with or without weights.

Pull-ups: This exercise targets the back, biceps, and shoulders. It can be performed with or without weights.

Shoulder press: This exercise targets the shoulders, triceps, and core. It can be performed with weights or resistance bands.

Bicep curls: This exercise targets the biceps and forearms. It can be performed with weights or resistance bands.

Planks: This exercise targets the core muscles. It can be performed with or without weights.

When designing a total body workout program that incorporates resistance training, it is important to consider the individual's fitness level, goals, and any physical limitations they may have. It is also important to vary the exercises and resistance used to prevent plateaus and boredom.

To see results from a total body workout program that incorporates resistance training, it is recommended to perform the exercises at least two to three times per week. It is also important to use proper form and technique to prevent injury and maximize the effectiveness of the exercises.

Moreover, resistance training can be done using different types of equipment, such as dumbbells, barbells, machines, resistance bands, or even bodyweight. Each type of equipment offers unique benefits and challenges, which can be used to vary the intensity and difficulty of the exercises. For example, free weights like dumbbells and barbells offer a greater range of motion and require more stabilization from the muscles, while machines provide more stability and control, making them ideal for beginners or those with joint issues.

In addition, resistance training can be done using different training techniques, such as high-intensity interval training (HIIT), supersets, drop sets, pyramid sets, and more. These techniques can be used to increase the intensity of the workouts, challenge the muscles in different ways, and promote muscle growth and strength gains.

Resistance training can also be customized to target specific muscle groups or areas of the body, depending on an individual's goals. For example, if someone wants to tone their arms, they can perform exercises like bicep curls, tricep dips, or lateral raises. If they want to strengthen their core, they can do exercises like planks, Russian twists, or crunches.

Furthermore, resistance training has been shown to offer many health benefits beyond muscle and strength gains. For example, it can help reduce the risk of injury by strengthening the muscles and bones, improve balance and coordination, enhance joint flexibility, and reduce inflammation in the body. Resistance training has also been shown to have a positive impact on mental health, by reducing stress and anxiety, improving mood and self-esteem, and promoting better sleep.

In summary, resistance training is a powerful tool for achieving a total body workout that targets multiple muscle groups and offers numerous health benefits. By incorporating a variety of exercises, equipment, and techniques, individuals can create a personalized workout program that suits their goals, fitness level, and preferences. Whether one wants to build muscle, tone their body, improve their health, or simply feel stronger and more confident, resistance training can help them achieve their goals

In conclusion, resistance training is a valuable component of a total body workout program. It provides numerous benefits for overall health and fitness and can be tailored to meet individual needs and goals. Incorporating a variety of resistance training exercises and performing them regularly with proper form and technique can help individuals achieve their desired results.

Proper form and technique in total body exercises

Proper form and technique are crucial components of total body exercises. These exercises are designed to work multiple muscle groups at once, making them efficient and effective. However, poor form and technique can lead to injury and reduce the effectiveness of the exercise. Therefore, it is essential to learn the proper form and technique for each exercise.

Before beginning any total body exercise, it is important to warm up properly. A good warm-up should include stretching and light cardio, such as jogging or jumping jacks. This will help increase blood flow and prepare the body for the workout.

When performing total body exercises, it is important to maintain proper posture. This means keeping your spine neutral, shoulders down and back, and core engaged. This will help prevent injury and ensure that the exercise is targeting the intended muscle groups.

One of the most common total body exercises is the squat. To perform a squat correctly, stand with your feet shoulder-width apart and toes pointing forward. Keep your chest up and engage your core. As you lower your body, push your hips back and down, keeping your knees in line with your toes. Go as low as you can without losing proper form, then push through your heels to stand back up. It is important to keep your weight in your heels and not let your knees go past your toes.

Another important total body exercise is the push-up. Start in a plank position with your hands slightly wider than shoulder-width apart. Keep your core engaged and lower your body down towards the ground, keeping your elbows close to your sides. Push back up to the starting position, keeping your body in a straight line throughout the movement. If this is too challenging, modify by performing the push-up from your knees.

The deadlift is another effective total body exercise. Begin with your feet shoulder-width apart and toes pointing forward. Hold a weight in front of your body, with your palms facing towards you. Keep your core engaged and hinge at your hips, lowering the weight down towards the ground. Keep your back straight and your weight in your heels. Once you feel a stretch in your hamstrings, drive through your heels to stand back up.

In conclusion, proper form and technique are crucial when performing total body exercises. By maintaining good posture, engaging your core, and using the correct form, you can prevent injury and ensure that the exercise is targeting the intended muscle groups. With consistent practice, you will see improvements in your strength and overall fitness.

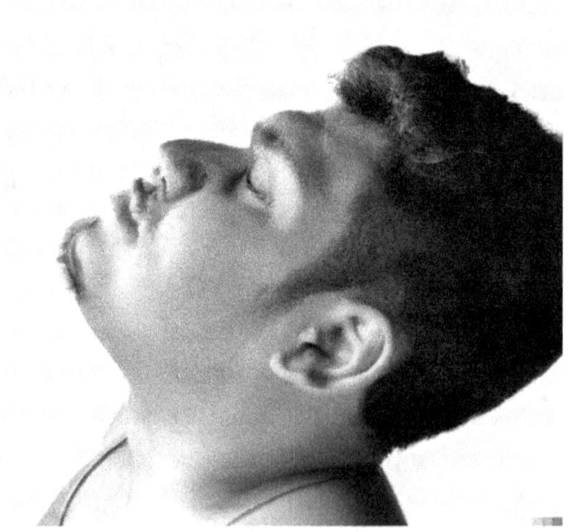

How to create a total body workout plan

Creating a total body workout plan can be a challenging task, especially for beginners who have little to no experience in designing a workout routine. However, with proper guidance and knowledge, it is possible to create a comprehensive and effective workout plan that targets all the major muscle groups in the body. Here are some steps to help you create a total body workout plan:

Step 1: Determine Your Fitness Goals

Before creating your workout plan, it is essential to determine your fitness goals. Your goals will determine the type of exercises you will include in your workout plan, the frequency, and the intensity of your workouts. Are you looking to build muscle, lose weight, or improve your overall fitness level? Once you have determined your fitness goals, you can begin to plan your workouts accordingly.

Step 2: Choose Your Exercises

The next step is to choose your exercises. A total body workout plan should include exercises that target all the major muscle groups, including the chest, back, legs, shoulders, arms, and core. Examples of exercises that can be included in your workout plan are squats, lunges, bench press, pull-ups, push-ups, deadlifts, and planks. It is also essential to include both resistance training and cardiovascular exercises to ensure that you are targeting all aspects of fitness.

Step 3: Determine the Number of Sets and Repetitions

Once you have chosen your exercises, it is time to determine the number of sets and repetitions for each exercise. The number of sets and reps will depend on your fitness goals, but a good starting point is to do three to four sets of each exercise, with 8-12 repetitions per set. This will help to build muscle and improve your overall fitness level.

Step 4: Plan Your Workouts

Now that you have chosen your exercises and determined the number of sets and reps, it is time to plan your workouts. It is important to schedule your workouts in advance and make sure that you are not overtraining any muscle group. For example, you could do upper body exercises one day and lower body exercises the next day to allow for adequate recovery time. It is also important to vary your workouts to prevent boredom and to challenge your body in different ways.

Step 5: Warm-Up and Cool-Down

Before beginning any workout, it is essential to warm up to prevent injury and prepare your body for exercise. A good warm-up should include five to ten minutes of light cardio, followed by stretching and mobility exercises. Similarly, cooling down after a workout is important to allow your body to recover. A good cool-down should include five to ten minutes of light cardio and stretching.

Step 6: Track Your Progress

It is essential to track your progress as you go through your total body workout plan. This can help you identify areas where you need to improve and make adjustments to your workout routine. Keeping a workout journal or using a fitness app can help you track your progress and see how far you have come.

Step 7: Adjust Your Workout Plan

As you progress through your workout plan, you may need to make adjustments to ensure that you continue to challenge yourself and see results. This can include increasing the weight you lift, adding new exercises to your routine, or changing the number of sets and reps you do. It is important to listen to your body and make adjustments as needed to avoid injury and achieve your fitness goals.

Step 8: Seek Professional Advice

If you are new to exercise or are unsure about how to create a total body workout plan, it is a good idea to seek professional advice. A personal trainer or fitness coach can help you create a workout plan that is tailored to your specific needs and fitness goals. They can also provide guidance on proper form and technique to prevent injury and ensure that you get the most out of your workouts.

In summary, creating a total body workout plan requires careful planning, dedication, and consistency. By following these steps, you can create an effective workout plan that targets all the major muscle groups in the body, helps you achieve your fitness goals, and improves your overall health and wellbeing. Remember to track your progress, make adjustments as needed, and seek professional advice if necessary.

In conclusion, creating a total body workout plan can be challenging, but with the right guidance and knowledge, it is possible to create an effective and comprehensive workout routine that targets all the major muscle groups in the body. By following these steps, you can create a workout plan that helps you achieve your fitness goals while improving your overall health and wellbeing.

The importance of rest and recovery in a total body workout

Rest and recovery are essential components of any effective total body workout. Although exercise is undoubtedly beneficial for overall health and fitness, it can also place a significant amount of stress on the body. During exercise, muscle fibers experience small amounts of damage and undergo micro-tears, which is a normal part of the muscle-building process. Rest and recovery allow the body to repair and rebuild these tissues, leading to increased strength and endurance.

One of the primary benefits of rest and recovery is the reduction of muscle soreness and fatigue. When you work out, lactic acid builds up in your muscles, leading to that familiar post-workout burn. Rest and recovery help to clear this lactic acid and other metabolic waste products from your muscles, reducing soreness and improving overall recovery.

Another benefit of rest and recovery is the prevention of overtraining. Overtraining occurs when you exercise too frequently or too intensely without allowing for adequate rest periods. This can lead to a decrease in performance, increased risk of injury, and overall fatigue. Rest and recovery help to prevent overtraining by allowing the body to fully recover between workouts and preventing the accumulation of fatigue over time.

Rest and recovery also play a critical role in injury prevention. When you work out, your muscles and joints are placed under significant stress. Without proper rest and recovery, this stress can lead to injury or strain. Rest and recovery allow the body to repair and rebuild tissues, reducing the risk of injury and improving overall physical health.

Lastly, rest and recovery can improve overall workout performance. When you give your body time to rest and recover, you allow your muscles to fully recharge and rebuild, leading to increased strength and endurance. Additionally, rest and recovery can help to improve focus and mental clarity, which can lead to better workout performance and more effective exercise.

There are various ways to incorporate rest and recovery into a total body workout program. One of the most effective ways is to alternate between different types of workouts. For example, if you are performing strength training exercises one day, you can do cardio or flexibility exercises on the next day. This allows your muscles to rest and recover while still maintaining your overall fitness.

Another important aspect of rest and recovery is sleep. During sleep, the body releases growth hormone, which is essential for tissue repair and rebuilding. Getting enough sleep is crucial to the body's recovery process and overall physical health. Aim for at least 7-8 hours of quality sleep per night to help your body recover and perform optimally.

Additionally, proper nutrition is essential for recovery after a workout. Adequate protein intake is important for muscle repair and growth, while carbohydrates are necessary to replenish glycogen stores in the muscles. Incorporating healthy fats, vitamins, and minerals into your diet can also support the body's recovery process.

It is also important to listen to your body and take rest days when necessary. If you feel excessively sore or fatigued, it may be a sign that your body needs rest. Taking a day off from exercise can help your muscles recover and prevent overtraining.

In summary, rest and recovery are critical components of any effective total body workout. By incorporating rest days, alternating between different types of workouts, getting enough sleep, eating a balanced diet, and listening to your body, you can ensure that you are giving your body the time and resources it needs to fully recover and perform at its best. Remember, a balanced approach to exercise that includes rest and recovery is key to achieving your overall health and fitness goals.

In conclusion, rest and recovery are essential components of any effective total body workout. By allowing the body to repair and rebuild tissues, reduce muscle soreness and fatigue, prevent overtraining and injury, and improve overall workout performance, rest and recovery play a critical role in achieving overall health and fitness goals. It is important to incorporate rest and recovery into any exercise program, to ensure that the body can fully benefit from the physical activity and avoid burnout or injury.

Nutrition and hydration for a total body workout

Nutrition and hydration are essential components of any total body workout regimen. Proper nutrition and hydration can help to maximize workout performance, support muscle growth and recovery, and prevent fatigue and injury. In this complex note, we will explore the importance of nutrition and hydration for a total body workout and provide recommendations for optimal intake.

Nutrition:

Before engaging in any total body workout, it is important to ensure that your body has the necessary fuel to perform at its best. This means consuming a balanced diet that includes a variety of macronutrients, including carbohydrates, proteins, and fats, as well as micronutrients such as vitamins and minerals. Each of these nutrients plays a unique role in supporting workout performance and recovery.

Carbohydrates: Carbohydrates are the primary fuel source for high-intensity exercise. They provide the body with the energy it needs to perform intense movements and maintain endurance. Consuming carbohydrates before and after a workout can help to replenish glycogen stores, which can enhance recovery and reduce fatigue.

Protein: Protein is essential for muscle growth and repair. When you engage in a total body workout, you are causing small tears in your muscle fibers. Protein helps to repair these tears and build new muscle tissue. Consuming protein before and after a workout can help to support muscle growth and recovery.

Fats: Fats are important for overall health and can provide a source of energy for lower-intensity exercise. They also help to support the absorption of fat-soluble vitamins, such as vitamin D.

Micronutrients: Micronutrients such as vitamins and minerals are essential for overall health and can help to support workout performance and recovery. For example, vitamin C can help to reduce muscle soreness, while iron is essential for transporting oxygen to the muscles.

Hydration:

Proper hydration is essential for optimal workout performance and recovery. When you engage in exercise, you lose fluids through sweat, and it is important to replace these fluids to prevent dehydration. Dehydration can lead to fatigue, muscle cramps, and reduced performance.

The American Council on Exercise recommends that individuals drink 17-20 ounces of fluid 2-3 hours before a workout and an additional 7-10 ounces every 10-20 minutes during the workout. Water is the best choice for hydration, but if you are engaging in a longer or more intense workout, you may also want to consider a sports drink that contains electrolytes.

Here are some examples of specific nutrition names that can be taken to support the above topics of nutrition and hydration for a total body workout:

Carbohydrates: Whole grain bread, brown rice, quinoa, sweet potatoes, fruits such as bananas and apples, and sports drinks containing carbohydrates.

Protein: Lean meats such as chicken and turkey, fish, beans, lentils, tofu, Greek yogurt, and protein supplements such as whey or casein protein powder.

Fats: Avocado, nuts, seeds, olive oil, salmon, and other fatty fish.

Micronutrients: Leafy green vegetables such as spinach and kale, citrus fruits such as oranges and grapefruits, nuts and seeds such as almonds and pumpkin seeds, and supplements such as vitamin C, vitamin D, and iron.

Hydration: Water, coconut water, sports drinks containing electrolytes, fruits and vegetables with high water content such as watermelon and cucumber, and herbal teas.

In addition to water and sports drinks, you can also hydrate through foods such as fruits and vegetables, which contain high levels of water. Some good options include watermelon, strawberries, cucumbers, and celery.

Conclusion, nutrition and hydration are essential components of any total body workout regimen. Consuming a balanced diet that includes carbohydrates, proteins, fats, and micronutrients can help to support workout performance and recovery. Proper hydration is also essential for preventing dehydration and optimizing workout performance. By paying attention to your nutrition and hydration, you can maximize the benefits of your total body workout and achieve your fitness goals.

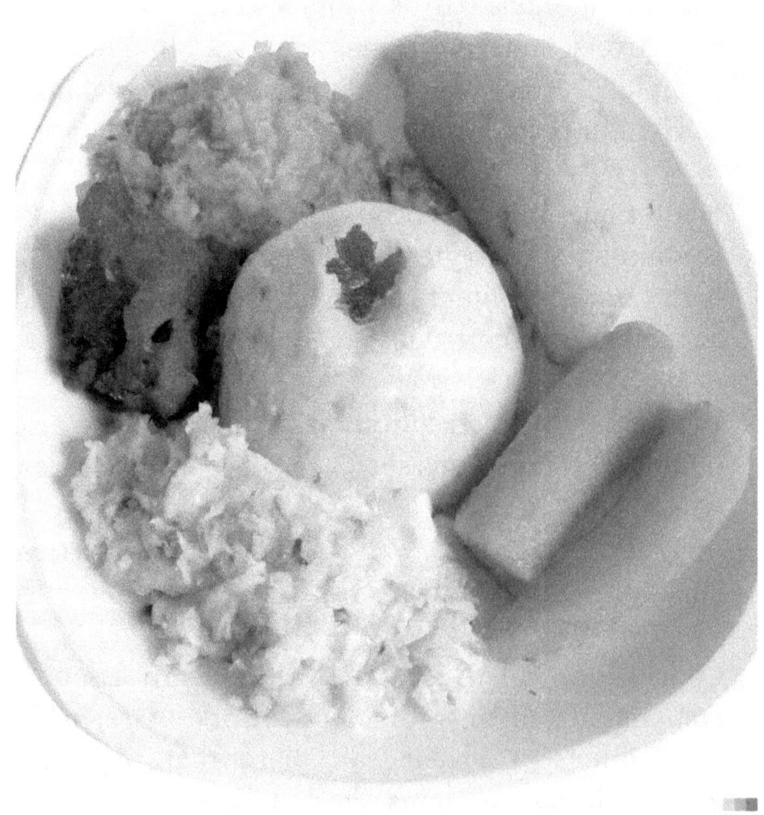

How to incorporate variety into a total body workout

Incorporating variety into a total body workout is an essential aspect of any effective exercise regimen. A varied workout routine not only helps prevent boredom but also ensures that all muscles are targeted, and the body is continually challenged. Here are some tips for incorporating variety into your total body workout.

Plan Your Workouts:
Planning your workouts in advance is an excellent way to incorporate variety. This means that you need to have a list of exercises that you want to do and a clear schedule for when you will do them. You can also change the order of the exercises each time you work out.

Use Different Equipment:
Using different equipment can add variety to your workouts. For instance, you can use resistance bands, free weights, or machines to perform different exercises. These different tools can work the same muscle groups but in different ways, ensuring that you target all muscle fibers.

Vary Your Reps and Sets:
Changing your reps and sets is an excellent way to add variety to your workouts. For instance, you can do high-rep, low-weight exercises one day and low-rep, high-weight exercises another day. You can also change the number of sets you perform to add variety to your workout.

Incorporate Cardio:
Cardiovascular exercise is an excellent way to add variety to your workouts. You can incorporate different types of cardio, such as running, cycling, or swimming, to keep your workouts fresh. Additionally, you can use different machines, such as the treadmill, elliptical, or stair climber, to change up your cardio routine.

Try Different Workouts:
Trying different workouts is an excellent way to incorporate variety into your total body workout. For instance, you can try Pilates, yoga, or kickboxing to challenge your body in different ways. You can also take a dance class or try a new sport to keep things exciting.

Mix Up Your Intensity:

Varying your intensity is an excellent way to add variety to your workouts. You can do high-intensity interval training (HIIT) one day and low-intensity steady-state cardio another day. Additionally, you can alternate between heavy lifting and bodyweight exercises to keep your workouts challenging.

Don't Forget About Rest:
Rest is an essential aspect of any workout regimen. Incorporating rest days into your schedule is an excellent way to allow your body to recover and prevent injury. Additionally, you can use active recovery, such as yoga or stretching, on your rest days to keep your body moving.

In conclusion, incorporating variety into your total body workout is essential for staying motivated and achieving your fitness goals. Planning your workouts, using different equipment, varying your reps and sets, incorporating cardio, trying different workouts, mixing up your intensity, and not forgetting about rest are all excellent ways to add variety to your workouts. Remember to listen to your body, challenge yourself, and have fun!

The role of stretching in a total body workout

Stretching is an essential component of any total body workout. It plays a vital role in preparing the body for exercise, preventing injuries, and enhancing overall flexibility and range of motion. In this article, we will explore the benefits of stretching and how it contributes to a complete workout routine.

Firstly, stretching helps to warm up the muscles and prepare them for physical activity. When you stretch, you increase blood flow to the muscles, which increases their temperature and makes them more pliable. This means that your muscles are better prepared to handle the stresses and strains of exercise. Proper stretching also helps to increase joint flexibility and range of motion, which makes it easier to perform exercises with good form.

In addition to warming up the muscles, stretching can help to prevent injuries during exercise. When your muscles are tight, they are more susceptible to injury, especially if you are performing exercises with a high degree of intensity or resistance. By stretching beforehand, you can help to loosen up your muscles, reduce the risk of strain, and prevent injuries from occurring.

Stretching also has many benefits for your overall health and well-being. It can help to reduce stress and tension in the muscles, which can alleviate pain and discomfort caused by sitting or standing for extended periods. Stretching can also help to improve posture, which can reduce the risk of back pain and other postural problems.

Moreover, stretching can be beneficial for those who engage in endurance activities such as running, cycling, or swimming. By improving your flexibility and range of motion, you can increase your stride length or improve your ability to reach further, which can lead to improved performance.

When incorporating stretching into your workout routine, it is essential to stretch all major muscle groups, including the hamstrings, quadriceps, calves, chest, back, shoulders, and neck. It is also crucial to stretch properly and safely, holding each stretch for 15-30 seconds and avoiding any bouncing or jerking movements.

Furthermore, stretching can also improve your balance and coordination, which can be beneficial for activities such as yoga or Pilates. By stretching regularly, you can improve your proprioception, which is your body's ability to sense its position and movement in space. This can help you to maintain your balance and stability during exercise, which can reduce the risk of falls or other accidents.

Another advantage of stretching is that it can help to reduce muscle soreness and stiffness after exercise. When you exercise, your muscles produce lactic acid, which can lead to soreness and fatigue. Stretching can help to flush out this lactic acid and other metabolic waste products, which can speed up the recovery process and reduce post-workout soreness.

Stretching can also be a form of relaxation and stress relief. When you stretch, you focus on your breath and your body, which can help to calm your mind and reduce feelings of anxiety or tension. This can be especially beneficial if you are feeling stressed or overwhelmed, as stretching can help you to release physical and emotional tension.

It is important to note that stretching should not be the only component of your workout routine. While stretching is beneficial for preparing the body for exercise and promoting flexibility, it is not sufficient for building strength or cardiovascular endurance. Therefore, it is important to include other forms of exercise, such as resistance training and cardiovascular activity, to achieve a complete workout.

In addition, stretching is an essential component of a total body workout. It helps to warm up the muscles, prevent injuries, promote flexibility and range of motion, improve balance and coordination, reduce muscle soreness and stiffness, and promote relaxation and stress relief. By incorporating stretching into your workout routine, you can enhance your overall fitness and well-being.

In conclusion, stretching plays a vital role in a total body workout. It helps to warm up the muscles, prevent injuries, and enhance overall flexibility and range of motion. By incorporating stretching into your workout routine, you can improve your performance, reduce the risk of injury, and promote overall health and well-being.

Tracking progress and setting goals in a total body workout

Tracking progress and setting goals in a total body workout is essential for achieving optimal fitness results. When you are engaged in a total body workout, it is crucial to focus on the right exercises, use the correct form and intensity, and keep track of your progress to ensure that you are making steady improvements towards your fitness goals. In this complex note, we will discuss various aspects of tracking progress and setting goals in a total body workout.

Setting Realistic Goals: The first step in tracking progress and achieving optimal results in a total body workout is to set realistic goals. You should consider your current fitness level, your desired outcomes, and your available resources, such as time and equipment. Set specific, measurable, and achievable goals that are aligned with your fitness objectives.

Tracking Progress: To track progress, you should establish a system to record your performance in each exercise or workout. This can be done by keeping a workout log or using a fitness app that records your progress. Your progress can be tracked by measuring the weight, reps, or time you spend on each exercise or workout. Tracking progress helps you identify areas where you are making progress and areas where you need to focus more effort.

Incorporating Variety: It is important to incorporate variety in your total body workout routine to prevent boredom and stimulate different muscle groups. You should include a mix of exercises that target different muscle groups, such as cardio, strength, and flexibility. Changing your routine every four to six weeks helps to avoid plateauing and ensures that you are challenging your body to continue making progress.

Balancing Workouts: You should balance your workouts by alternating between strength and cardio exercises. Strength exercises help to build muscle and increase metabolism, while cardio exercises help to burn calories and improve cardiovascular health. Balancing your workouts ensures that you are getting a full-body workout and achieving optimal fitness results.

Adapting to Challenges: In a total body workout, you will encounter challenges, such as injuries, lack of motivation, or a busy schedule. It is important to adapt to these challenges and adjust your workout routine accordingly. You should seek professional advice if you are injured, find ways to motivate yourself, and modify your workout routine to fit your schedule.

Celebrating Achievements: Finally, you should celebrate your achievements along the way. Celebrating small wins, such as an increase in reps or weight lifted, helps to keep you motivated and focused on your goals. You can also reward yourself with non-food rewards, such as a massage or a new workout outfit, when you reach significant milestones.

In conclusion, tracking progress and setting goals in a total body workout is essential for achieving optimal fitness results. By setting realistic goals, tracking progress, incorporating variety, balancing workouts, adapting to challenges, and celebrating achievements, you can ensure that you are making steady improvements towards your fitness objectives. Remember, consistency and dedication are key to achieving your fitness goals.

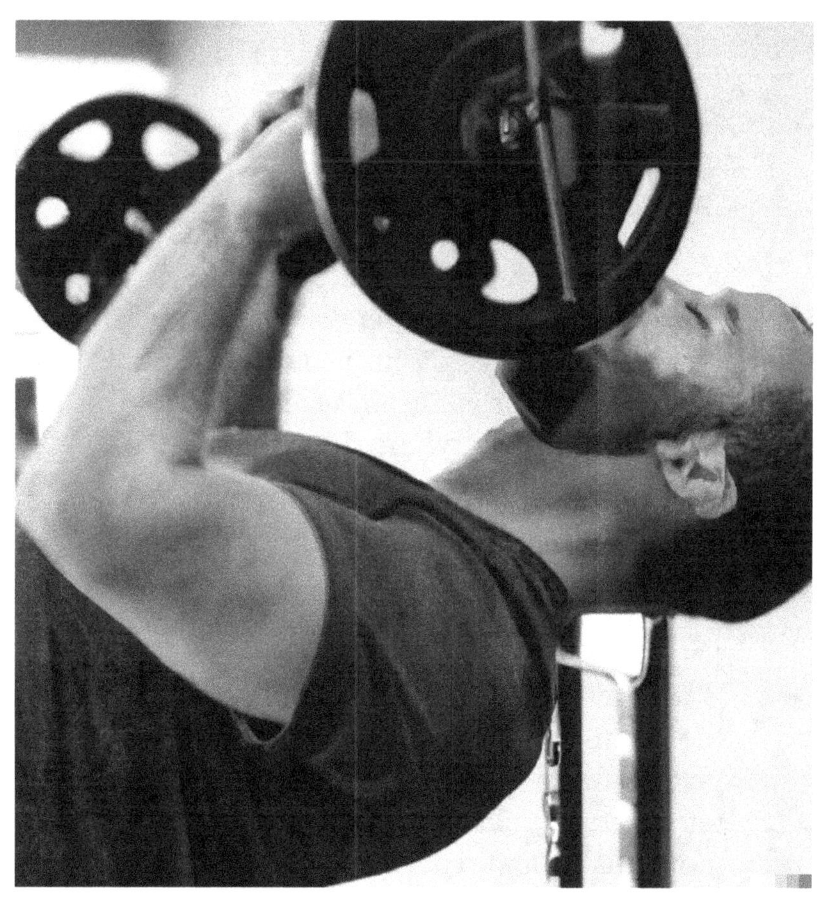

Avoiding common mistakes in a total body workout

A total body workout is an excellent way to get in shape and achieve overall health and fitness. However, it's essential to avoid common mistakes that can prevent you from reaching your goals and even lead to injury. In this complex note, we'll discuss some of the most common mistakes people make when doing a total body workout and how to avoid them.

Lack of Proper Warm-up
One of the biggest mistakes people make is skipping the warm-up before starting a total body workout. A proper warm-up helps increase blood flow, body temperature, and flexibility, making your muscles more pliable and reducing the risk of injury. A good warm-up should consist of low-intensity cardio, stretching, and mobility exercises.

Overtraining
Overtraining is a common mistake people make when they first start a total body workout. They believe that working out more frequently or for longer durations will yield better results. However,

overtraining can lead to injuries, burnout, and a lack of progress. It's important to find the right balance between workout intensity, frequency, and duration to avoid overtraining.

Neglecting Compound Movements

Compound movements, such as squats, deadlifts, and bench presses, are the foundation of any total body workout. They work multiple muscle groups simultaneously, helping you build overall strength and muscle mass. Neglecting compound movements in favor of isolation exercises can limit your progress and lead to muscle imbalances.

Not Using Proper Form

Using proper form is crucial when doing any exercise, but especially when doing a total body workout. Poor form can lead to injury, and it can also limit your progress by preventing you from engaging the correct muscles. Take the time to learn proper form for each exercise and use a weight that allows you to perform the exercise with good form.

Ignoring Rest and Recovery

Rest and recovery are essential for making progress in a total body workout. When you work out, you're breaking down muscle tissue, and it's during rest and recovery that your muscles rebuild and grow stronger. Ignoring rest and recovery can lead to overtraining, burnout, and a lack of progress. Make sure to incorporate rest days into your workout schedule and prioritize sleep and proper nutrition.

Not Varying Your Workouts
Finally, not varying your workouts can lead to plateaus in progress and boredom. Your body adapts quickly to exercise, and doing the same routine week after week can limit your progress. Make sure to vary your workouts by changing up the exercises, weights, reps, and sets to keep your body guessing and challenged.

Focusing Too Much on Cardio
Cardiovascular exercise is an essential component of any workout routine, but it's important not to focus too much on cardio at the expense of strength training. While cardio is great for burning calories and improving cardiovascular health, strength training is essential for building muscle, improving bone density, and boosting metabolism. Make sure to include both strength training and cardio in your total body workout routine.

Skipping Recovery Days
It's tempting to push yourself hard every day, especially when you're motivated and eager to see

results. However, it's important to give your body time to recover and repair itself between workouts. Skipping recovery days can lead to fatigue, burnout, and injury. Make sure to incorporate rest days into your workout routine and prioritize sleep and recovery.

Neglecting Flexibility Training

Flexibility training is often overlooked in total body workout routines, but it's crucial for improving range of motion, reducing the risk of injury, and preventing muscle imbalances. Incorporate stretching and mobility exercises into your warm-up and cooldown routines to improve flexibility and mobility.

Not Listening to Your Body

Perhaps the most significant mistake you can make in a total body workout routine is not listening to your body. Pushing yourself too hard or ignoring pain or discomfort can lead to injury and setbacks. Pay attention to how your body feels and adjust your workout intensity or routine as needed. It's better to take a step back and rest or modify your routine than to risk injury or burnout.

In conclusion, a total body workout can be an effective way to achieve overall health and fitness, but it's important to avoid common mistakes. Make sure to warm up properly, find the right balance between workout intensity and rest, incorporate compound movements, use proper form, and vary your workouts to keep your body challenged. With these tips, you can avoid common mistakes and make progress toward your fitness goals.

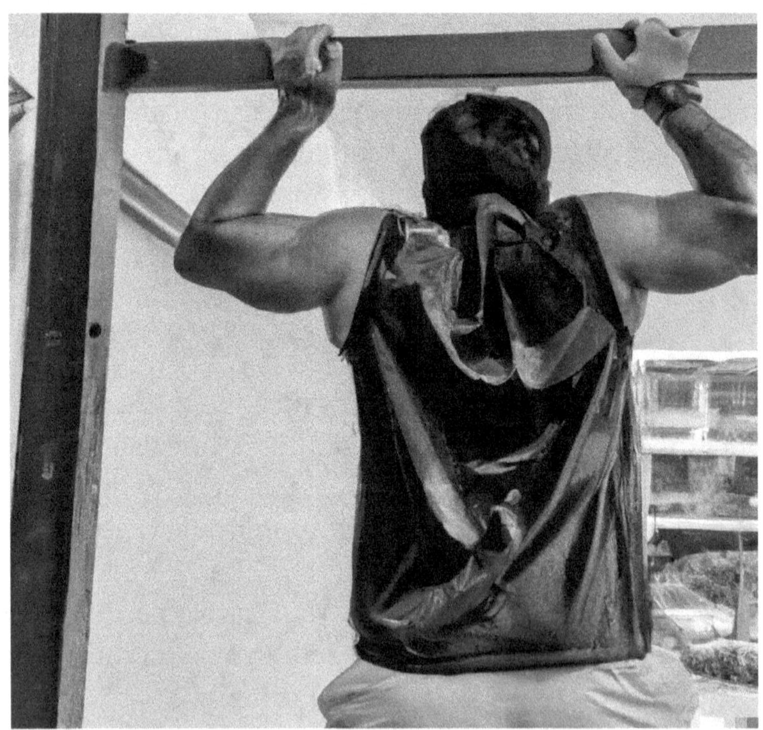

Incorporating total body workouts into your daily routine

Incorporating total body workouts into your daily routine can have numerous benefits for your overall health and well-being. Total body workouts involve exercises that engage multiple muscle groups simultaneously, leading to increased calorie burn and improved muscular endurance, strength, and cardiovascular health. However, it is important to approach total body workouts with care, as they can be physically demanding and require proper form to avoid injury.

One approach to incorporating total body workouts into your daily routine is to start with a balanced workout plan that includes a variety of exercises that target different muscle groups. This can include compound exercises, such as squats, lunges, and push-ups, which engage multiple muscle groups at once. Other exercises that target specific muscle groups, such as bicep curls and tricep extensions, can also be included.

To get the most out of your total body workout, it is important to focus on proper form and technique. This means engaging your core muscles and maintaining a neutral spine throughout each exercise. Additionally, you should be mindful of your breathing, inhaling as you lower the weight and exhaling as you lift it.

When it comes to scheduling your total body workouts, there are a few options to consider. You may choose to perform a full-body workout two to three times per week, with a day of rest in between to allow for muscle recovery. Alternatively, you may opt for split workouts, where you focus on upper body exercises one day and lower body exercises the next. This can help to reduce muscle fatigue and allow for greater intensity during each workout.

It is also important to remember that total body workouts can be modified to fit your individual needs and fitness level. This may involve adjusting the amount of weight used, the number of reps performed, or the rest periods between sets. Consulting with a personal trainer or fitness professional can help you to develop a workout plan that is tailored to your specific goals and needs.

Incorporating total body workouts into your daily routine can provide a number of benefits, including improved muscular endurance, strength, and cardiovascular health. However, it is important to approach these workouts with care, focusing on proper form and technique, and adjusting the intensity to fit your individual needs. By following these guidelines, you can develop a workout plan that supports your overall health and well-being.

How to stay motivated in a total body workout.

Motivation is a key factor in achieving any fitness goal, and staying motivated throughout a total body workout can be particularly challenging. However, there are several strategies that can help you stay motivated and committed to your fitness routine.

Set clear goals: One of the most important factors in staying motivated during a total body workout is having clear, specific goals. Define what you want to achieve, such as losing weight, building muscle, or improving your cardiovascular fitness, and then set achievable targets for each goal. Having clear goals will help you stay focused and motivated, and will give you a sense of accomplishment as you progress.

Mix up your routine: Doing the same workout day in and day out can quickly become monotonous and lead to a lack of motivation. To keep things interesting, try incorporating different types of workouts into your routine, such as strength training, cardio, and flexibility exercises. You can also switch up the order of your exercises, vary the number of reps or sets, or try different equipment.

Track your progress: Keeping track of your progress is a great way to stay motivated and see how far you've come. Use a fitness app or journal to record your workouts, track your weight, and measure your body fat percentage. Seeing progress in these metrics can be a powerful motivator, and can help you stay on track when you're feeling discouraged.

Find a workout partner: Working out with a friend or family member can be a great way to stay motivated and accountable. Having someone to push you and cheer you on can make all the difference when you're feeling tired or unmotivated. Plus, it's a great way to socialize and stay connected with others.

Reward yourself: Finally, don't forget to reward yourself for your hard work and dedication. Set up a reward system for yourself, such as treating yourself to a massage or a new workout outfit when you hit a certain goal. Celebrating your accomplishments can help you stay motivated and focused on your fitness goals.

Have a positive mindset: Maintaining a positive mindset is crucial for staying motivated during a total body workout. Negative self-talk and thoughts of self-doubt can quickly undermine your motivation and make it harder to stay committed. Instead, focus on positive self-talk and remind yourself of your goals and why you started your fitness journey in the first place.

Take rest days: Rest days are just as important as workout days. Overtraining can lead to fatigue, burnout, and injuries, which can all dampen your motivation. Incorporating rest days into your workout routine will help you avoid burnout, allow your muscles to recover, and give you the energy and motivation to tackle your next workout.

Create a supportive environment: Having a supportive environment can help you stay motivated and committed to your fitness routine. Surround yourself with people who share your goals and values, and who encourage and motivate you to achieve your best. You can also create a supportive environment by listening to motivating music, watching inspirational videos, or reading fitness blogs or books.

Keep it fun: If you're not enjoying your workout, it can be hard to stay motivated. Try to find ways to make your workout fun and enjoyable, such as listening to music, working out outdoors, or trying new exercises or equipment. Experiment with different workouts and find what works best for you.

Embrace the journey: Remember that your fitness journey is a marathon, not a sprint. There will be ups and downs, setbacks and breakthroughs, but staying committed and motivated throughout the journey will ultimately lead to success. Embrace the process, stay patient, and keep pushing yourself to be your best.

Overall, staying motivated during a total body workout requires dedication, focus, and a willingness to try new things. By setting clear goals, mixing up your routine, tracking your progress, finding a workout partner, and rewarding yourself, you can stay motivated and committed to achieving your fitness goals.